POWER OF PREVENTION

How to Beat Back Disease and Live a Long, Healthy Life.

Joseph Rutherford

TERMS OF USE

This book is for personal use only. Do not sell, distribute, or modify this book without the express written permission of the author. **Connect with the Author at:**

www.josephrutherford.com

ojosephrutherford@gmail.com

DISCLAIMER

While creating this book, the author strived to be as accurate and complete as possible, including information from a variety of sources, including medical journals, government websites, and reputable health organizations. The author is a Behavioral Change Communicator and does not claim to be able to diagnose or treat any medical conditions. If you have any concerns about your health, please consult with a doctor or other qualified healthcare provider. The information in this book is not a substitute for a doctor's diagnosis or treatment. Note that what worked for some people may not work for others. Following the advice found in this book may result in unintended consequences which the author assumes no responsibility for. Application of the advice herein are solely at the risk of the reader. Always consult with your doctor or other qualified healthcare provider before making any changes to your diet, exercise routine, or other aspects of your health.

DEDICATION

This book is dedicated to Goodness Rutherford, Jayden Rutherford Silas, and to all the professionals who are working to prevent disease and improve health.

Your work is essential to our well-being. You are the ones who help us make healthy choices, stay informed about our health, and get the care we need.

Thank you for all that you do.

Specifically, I would like to thank the following professionals:

The doctors, nurses, and other healthcare providers who care for us.

The researchers who are working to find new ways to prevent disease and improve health.

The public health officials who are working to make our communities healthier.

The educators who are teaching us about health and wellness.

I am grateful for your dedication and commitment to making the world a healthier place.

CONTENTS

Chapter 3: Stress Management

The importance of stress management

How to manage stress

Chapter 4: Sleep

The importance of sleep

The effects of sleep deprivation

Tips to get a good night sleep

Chapter 5: Drink Water

Water can help prevent health problems

Water can help to improve our overall health and well-being

Recommended daily water intake

Water drinking tips

Chapter 6: Other Lifestyle Factors

Smoking

Alcohol use

Sun exposure

Weight management

Tips for managing lifestyle factors that affect your health

Chapter 7: Screening Tests

Benefits of screening tests

The risks of screening tests

Common screening test recommended for adults

Chapter 8: Pyramid Energy Mat

What is Pyramid Energy Mat?

How does it work

Effects of using Pyramid Energy Mat

PREFACE

As we age, our chances of developing long-term health issues tend to rise. This is because our bodies become less resilient and more susceptible to disease. However, there are many things we can do to prevent these illnesses.

Prevention is the key to good health. By making healthy choices today, we can help ensure a healthy future for ourselves and our loved ones.

This book is designed to help you learn more about prevention. It covers a variety of topics, including diet and nutrition, exercise, stress management, sleep, and other lifestyle factors. It also discusses the importance of screening tests and how to take control of your health.

I hope this book will help you understand the importance of prevention and to take steps to improve your health. You can live a long, healthy, and happy life by making healthy choices and caring for yourself.

I hope you find this book helpful. Please let me know if you have any questions.

Sincerely,

Joseph Rutherford

INTRODUCTION

T he likelihood of developing chronic health conditions is higher from age 40 and beyond. However, there are many things we can do to prevent these conditions from developing or slowing their progression, and this is where prevention comes in.

WHAT IS PREVENTION?

Prevention is avoiding or reducing the risk of developing a disease or condition. There are many different types of prevention, including:

Primary Prevention: This is the prevention of disease before it starts. Examples of primary prevention include eating a healthy diet, exercising regularly, and getting enough sleep.

Secondary Prevention: This is the early detection and treatment of a disease to prevent it from becoming more serious. Examples of secondary prevention include screening tests for cancer and other diseases and taking medications to control chronic conditions.

Tertiary Prevention: This prevents further complications from a disease already diagnosed. Examples of tertiary prevention include rehabilitation after a stroke or heart attack and managing chronic conditions to prevent them from worsening.

WHY IS PREVENTION IMPORTANT?

Prevention is vital for everyone, but it is essential for people in midlife and beyond because as we age, our chances of developing long-term health issues tend to rise as we age. One of the best ways to improve our chances of living a satisfying and healthy life is to proactively work toward preventing these illnesses.

COMMON HEALTH ISSUES IN MIDLIFE AND BEYOND

Cardiovascular disease: This is the leading cause of death, and it is more common in people as they get older. There are many risk factors for cardiovascular disease, including high blood pressure, high cholesterol, smoking, and obesity.

Cancer: Cancer is another leading cause of death worldwide, and it can strike at any age. However, the risk of cancer increases as people get older. Some of the most common types of cancer in midlife and beyond include breast cancer, prostate cancer, lung cancer, and colon cancer.

Diabetes: Diabetes is a chronic disease that affects the way your body turns food into energy. There are two main types of diabetes: type 1 and type 2. Type 1 diabetes is an autoimmune disease, and it usually develops in childhood or adolescence. Type 2 diabetes is more common, and it is usually caused by a combination of genetics and lifestyle factors such as obesity and physical inactivity.

Arthritis: Arthritis is a condition that causes pain and inflammation in the joints. There are many different types of arthritis, and the most common type in midlife and beyond is osteoarthritis. Osteoarthritis is caused by wear and tear on the joints, and it is more common in people who are overweight or obese.

Osteoporosis: Osteoporosis is a condition that causes bones to become weak and brittle. It is more common in women than men, and the risk increases as people get older. Osteoporosis can lead to fractures, especially in the hip, spine, and wrist.

Depression: Depression is a common mental health disorder that can affect people at any age. However, the risk of depression increases as people get older. Depression can cause a variety of symptoms, including sadness, fatigue, changes in appetite, and difficulty sleeping.

Cognitive decline: Cognitive decline is a gradual decline in mental abilities such as memory, thinking, and judgment. It is a normal part of aging, but it can also be a sign of a more serious condition such as Alzheimer's disease.

It is important to see your doctor regularly if you are in midlife or beyond. This will help to ensure that you are getting the care you need to stay healthy. If you have any concerns about your health, be sure to talk to your doctor.

In this book, we will discuss the importance of prevention and how you can take steps to prevent common health problems in midlife and beyond. We will cover various topics, including diet and nutrition, exercise, stress management, sleep, and other lifestyle factors. We will also discuss the importance of screening tests and how to take control of your health.

This book will help you to understand the importance of prevention and will guide you on steps to improve your health. You can live a long, healthy, and happy life by making healthy choices and caring for yourself and your loved ones.

CHAPTER 1: DIET AND NUTRITION

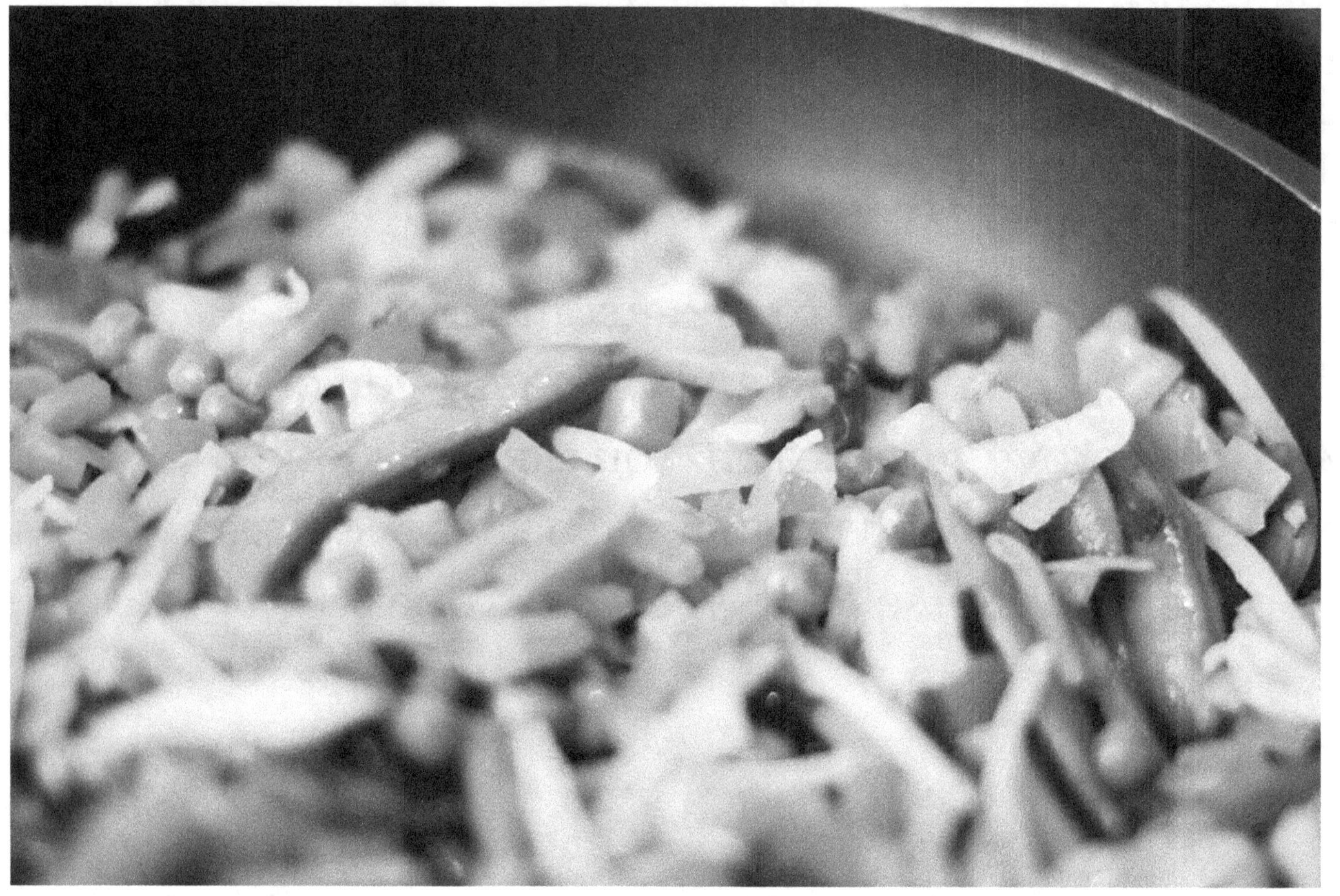

THE IMPORTANCE OF EATING A HEALTHY DIET

Eating a healthy diet is essential for good health. It can help you maintain a healthy weight, reduce your risk of chronic diseases, and improve your overall well-being.

A healthy diet includes a variety of nutrient-rich foods from all food groups, which means eating plenty of fruits, vegetables, whole grains, lean protein, and healthy fats. It is also important to limit your intake of processed foods, sugary drinks, and unhealthy fats.

These are a few reasons why it is important to limit your intake of them:

Processed foods

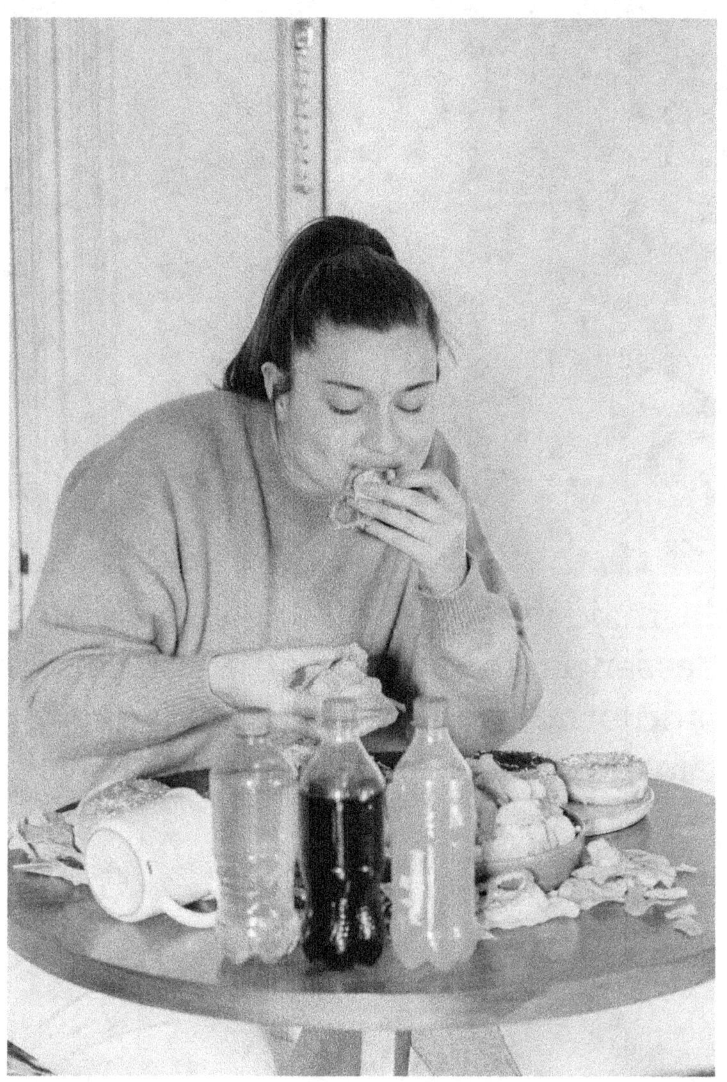

Many processed foods tend to contain a lot of unhealthy fats, added sugars, and sodium. They may also contain artificial ingredients and preservatives. These foods can contribute to weight gain, heart disease, and other health problems. Processed foods are often high in calories and low in nutrients. They may also contain artificial ingredients and preservatives that have not been well-studied.

Sugary drinks

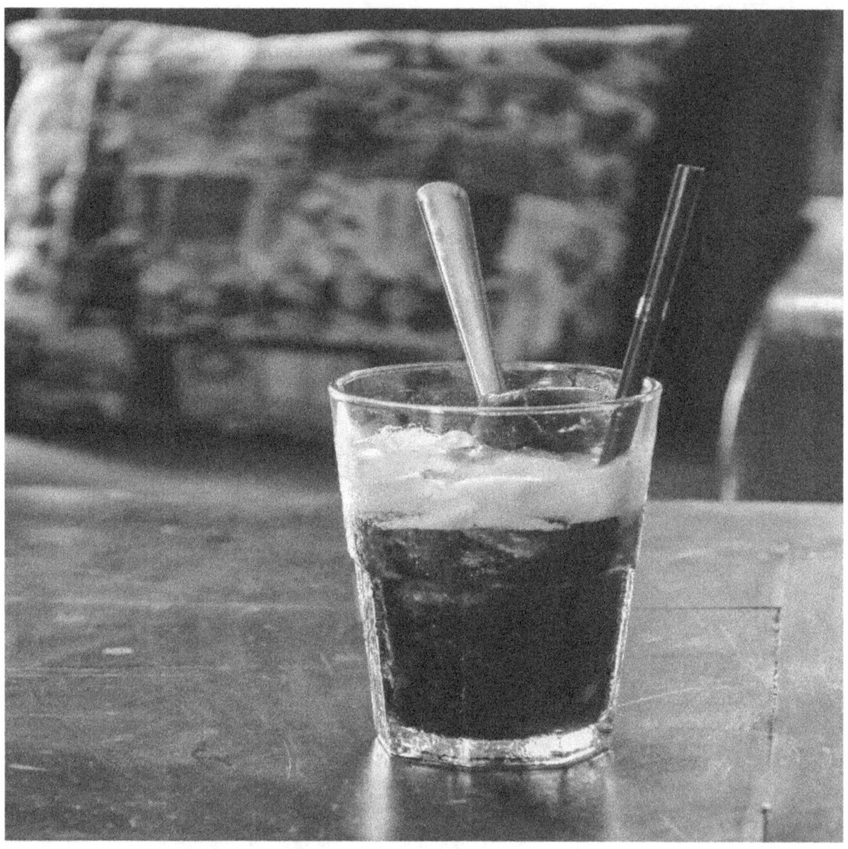

Sugary drinks are a major source of added sugar in the American diet. Added sugar is not essential for good health and can contribute to weight gain, tooth decay, and other health problems. Sugary drinks are a major source of empty calories. They can contribute to weight gain and tooth decay.

Unhealthy fats

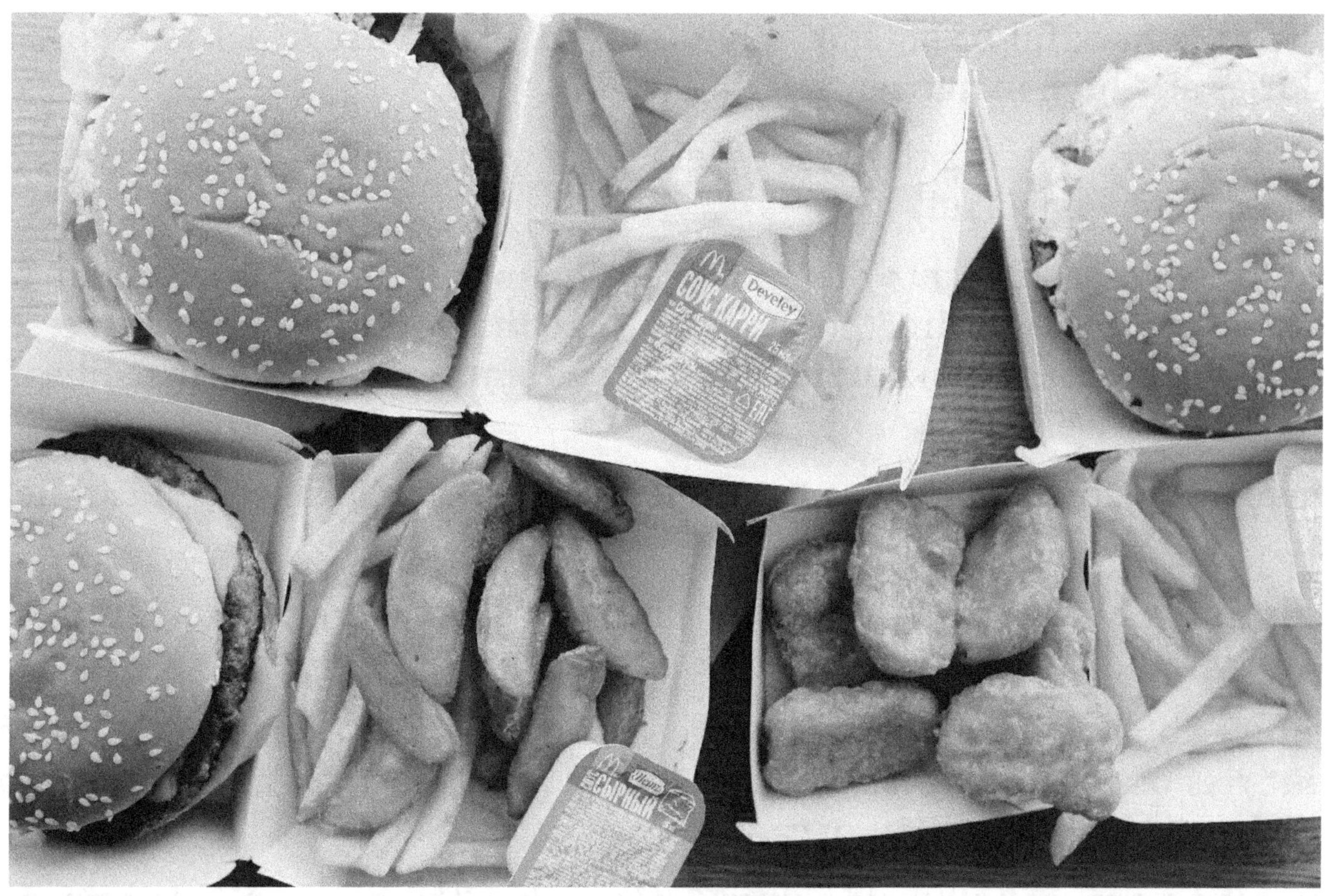

Unhealthy fats, such as saturated and trans fats, can increase your risk of heart disease. They can also contribute to weight gain. Unhealthy fats can increase your risk of heart disease, stroke, and some types of cancer.

If you are looking to improve your diet, it is important to limit your intake of processed foods, sugary drinks, and unhealthy fats. Instead, focus on eating whole, unprocessed foods that are high in nutrients. These foods will help you feel full and satisfied, and they will also provide your body with the nutrients it needs to stay healthy.

Here are some tips for limiting your intake of these foods:

Read food labels: When you are shopping for food, be sure to read the food labels carefully. Look for foods that are low in calories, fat, and added sugar.

Cook at home: Cooking at home gives you more control over the ingredients in your food. When you cook at home, you can avoid processed foods and sugary drinks.

Make healthy snacks: If you are looking for a snack, reach for a piece of fruit, a handful of nuts, or a hard-boiled egg. These snacks are low in calories and high in nutrients.

Drink water: Water is the best beverage for your health. It is calorie-free, and it helps you feel full.

Making changes to your diet can seem daunting, but it is worth it for your health. By following these tips, you can limit your intake of processed foods, sugary drinks, and unhealthy fats and start enjoying the benefits of a healthy lifestyle.

There are many benefits to eating a healthy diet. For example, it can help you:

Maintain a healthy weight: Eating a healthy diet can help you maintain a healthy weight or lose weight if you are overweight or obese.

Reduce your risk of chronic diseases: Eating a healthy diet can help reduce your risk of developing chronic diseases such as heart disease, stroke, type 2 diabetes, and some types of cancer.

Improve your overall well-being: Eating a healthy diet can help improve your energy levels, mood, and sleep quality. It can also help boost your immune system and protect you from infections.

THE MEDITERRANEAN DIET

The Mediterranean diet comprises traditional foods from the Mediterranean region and is known for its health benefits. This diet contains fruits, vegetables, whole grains, legumes, nuts, and seeds. The diet comprises reasonable portions of fish, poultry, and dairy items.

The Mediterranean diet is a great way to improve your health, offering numerous benefits such as:

- Reducing the risk of heart disease
- Reducing the risk of stroke
- Reducing the risk of type 2 diabetes
- Lowering the likelihood of developing certain forms of cancer.
- Improving cognitive function
- Increasing lifespan

THE DASH DIET

The DASH diet is another healthy diet designed to help lower blood pressure consisting of low-fat dairy products, rich in vegetables, fruits, and whole grains. Eating lean protein and healthy fats is also important but in moderation.

The DASH diet has proven to be successful in reducing blood pressure levels, and it could potentially offer additional health advantages, including minimizing the likelihood of heart disease and stroke.

HOW TO MAKE HEALTHY FOOD CHOICES

There are many other healthy diets that you can follow. Some popular options include the vegan diet, the vegetarian diet, and the gluten-free diet.

The best diet for you will depend on your individual needs and preferences. Suppose you still need to determine which diet is proper. Discuss it with your physician or a certified dietitian in that case.

There are a few simple things you can do to make healthy food choices:

Read food labels carefully.

Select foods low in trans fat, saturated fat, and sodium.

Opt for foods high in fiber, fruits, vegetables, and whole grains.

- Limit your processed foods, sugary drinks, and red meat intake.

Tips for Eating Healthy

Here are a few tips for eating healthy:

- Plan your meals ahead of time.
- Cook at home more often.
- Pack your lunches and snacks.
- Eat breakfast every day.
- Make healthy choices when you eat out.

Conclusion

Maintaining a nutritious diet is crucial for improving your overall well-being. By following the tips in this chapter, you can significantly improve your overall health while also reducing the risk of chronic diseases. It's important to prioritize a nutritious diet by choosing healthy beverage options and food consumption. By doing so, you can take a proactive approach to your well-being and ensure that you're doing everything in your power to stay healthy.

CHAPTER 2: EXERCISE

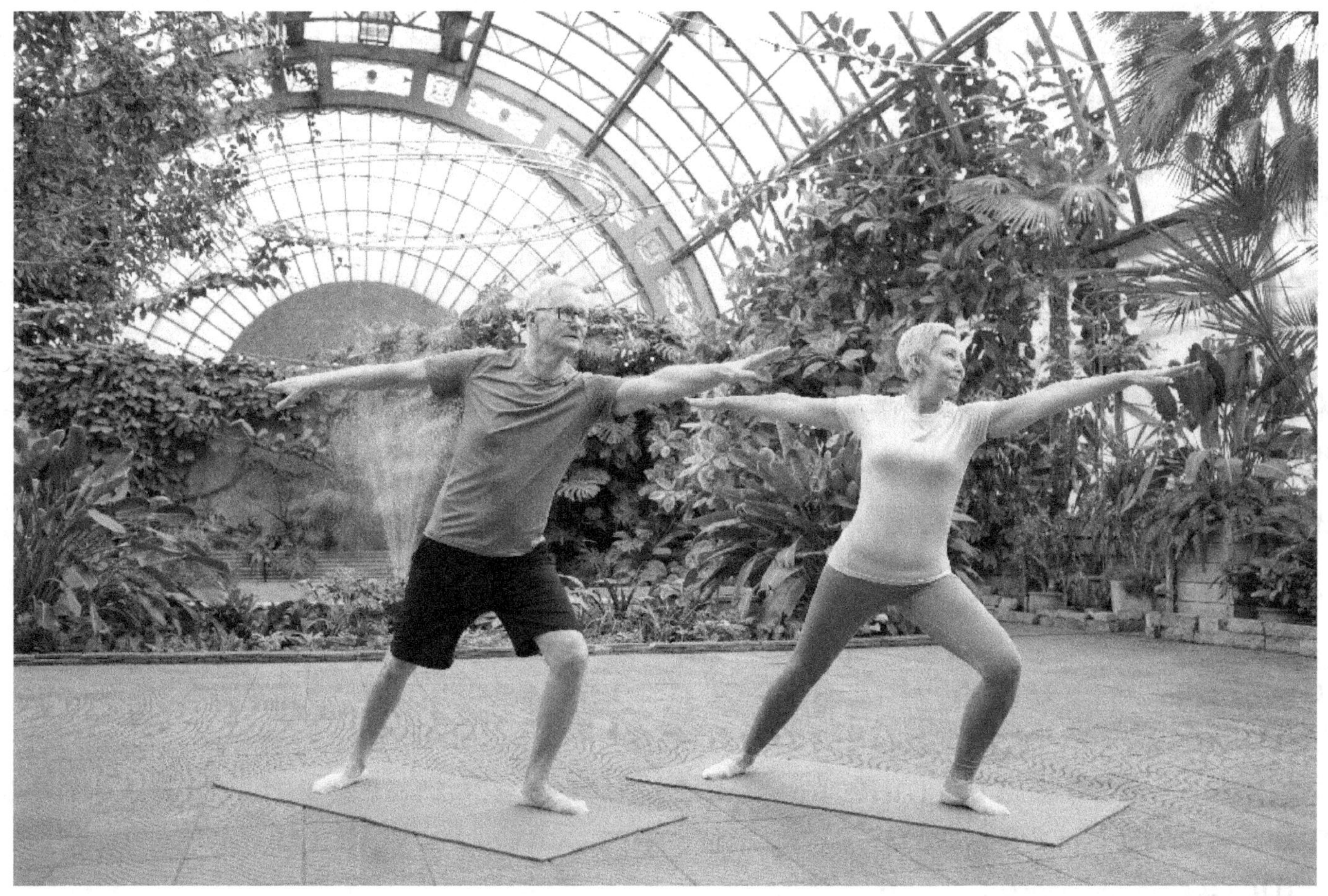

THE IMPORTANCE OF EXERCISE

Exercise is important for people of all ages, but it is especially important for people in midlife and beyond. As we age, our bodies become less active, and this can lead to a number of health problems. Exercise can help to prevent these problems and improve overall health and well-being.

Incorporating exercise into your daily routine is essential for maintaining a healthy lifestyle. Regular physical activity can aid in weight management, lower the likelihood of developing chronic illnesses, and enhance overall well-being.

THE BENEFITS OF EXERCISE

Regular exercise can decrease the likelihood of chronic diseases such as heart disease, stroke, type 2 diabetes, and certain types of cancer and other chronic diseases.

Improves mental health: Exercise can help improve mood, reduce stress, and boost self-esteem.

Increases energy levels: Exercise can help you feel more energetic throughout the day.

Strengthens bones and muscles: Exercise can help keep your bones and muscles strong and healthy.

Improves balance and coordination: Exercise can help improve your balance and coordination, which can help prevent falls.

Helps you sleep better: Exercise can help you sleep better at night.

HOW MUCH EXERCISE DO YOU NEED?

The Centers for Disease Control and Prevention (CDC) recommends that adults get at least 150 minutes of moderate-intensity aerobic activity or 75 minutes of vigorous-intensity aerobic exercise each week. They also suggest that adults do muscle-strengthening activities that work all major muscle groups (legs, hips, back, abdomen, chest, shoulders, and arms) two or more days a week.

FINDING AN EXERCISE ROUTINE THAT WORKS FOR YOU

The best way to find an exercise routine that works for you is to experiment with different activities and find ones you enjoy. You should also ensure that your practice is manageable. If you are new to exercise, gradually increase your workouts' intensity and duration.

TIPS FOR GETTING STARTED WITH EXERCISE

Here are a few tips for getting started with exercise:

Set realistic goals: Only attempt to do a little at a time. Start with small goals and gradually increase them as you get fitter.

Find an exercise buddy: Exercising with a friend or family member can help you stay motivated.

Make it fun: Choose activities that you enjoy and that fit into your lifestyle.

Be bold and ask for help: If you need help getting started, talk to your doctor or a certified personal trainer.

TYPES OF EXERCISE

There are many different types of exercise that you can do. Some popular options include:

Aerobic exercise

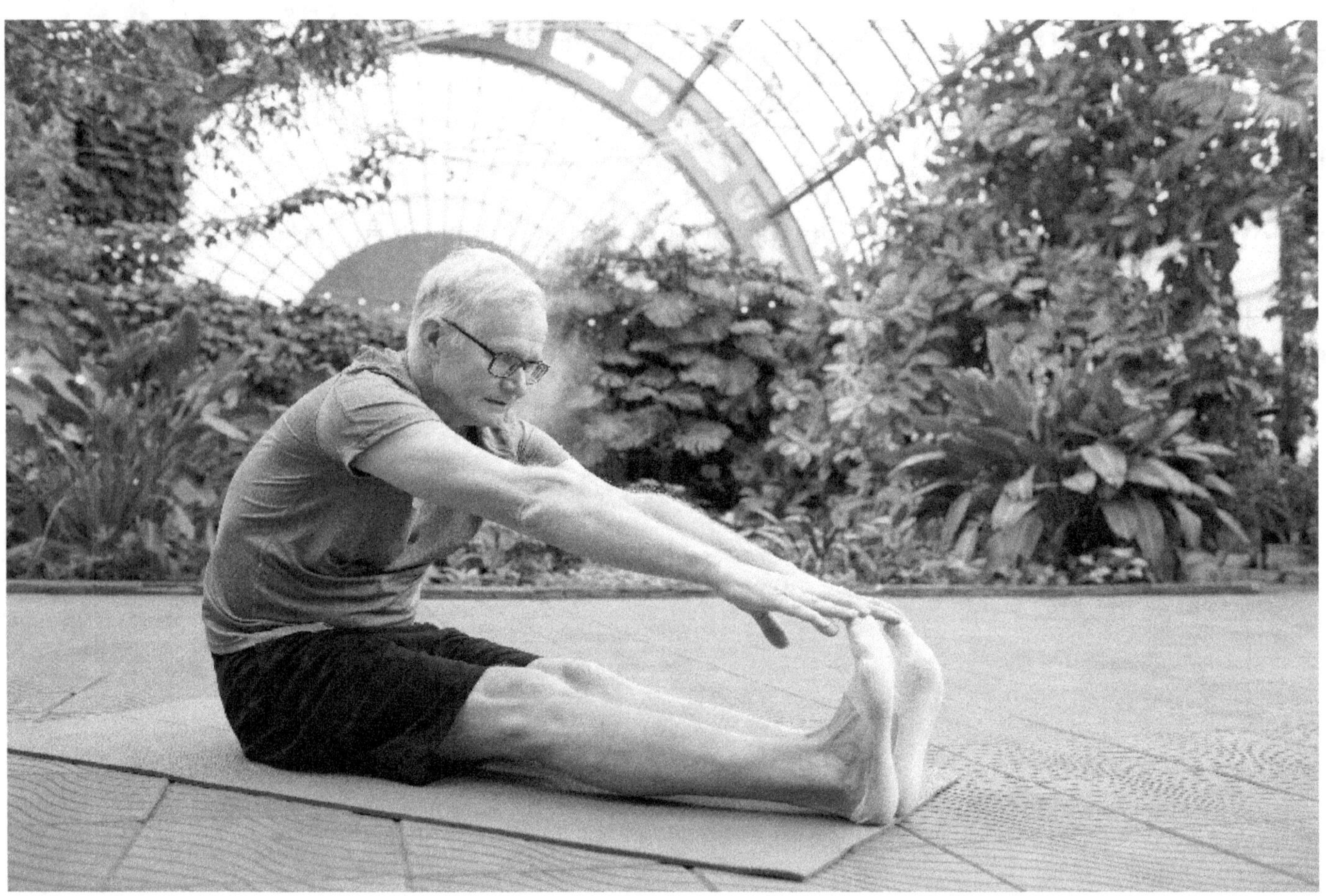

This exercise increases your heart rate and blood flow. Aerobic exercise includes walking, running, biking, swimming, dancing, and jumping rope.

Strength-training exercise

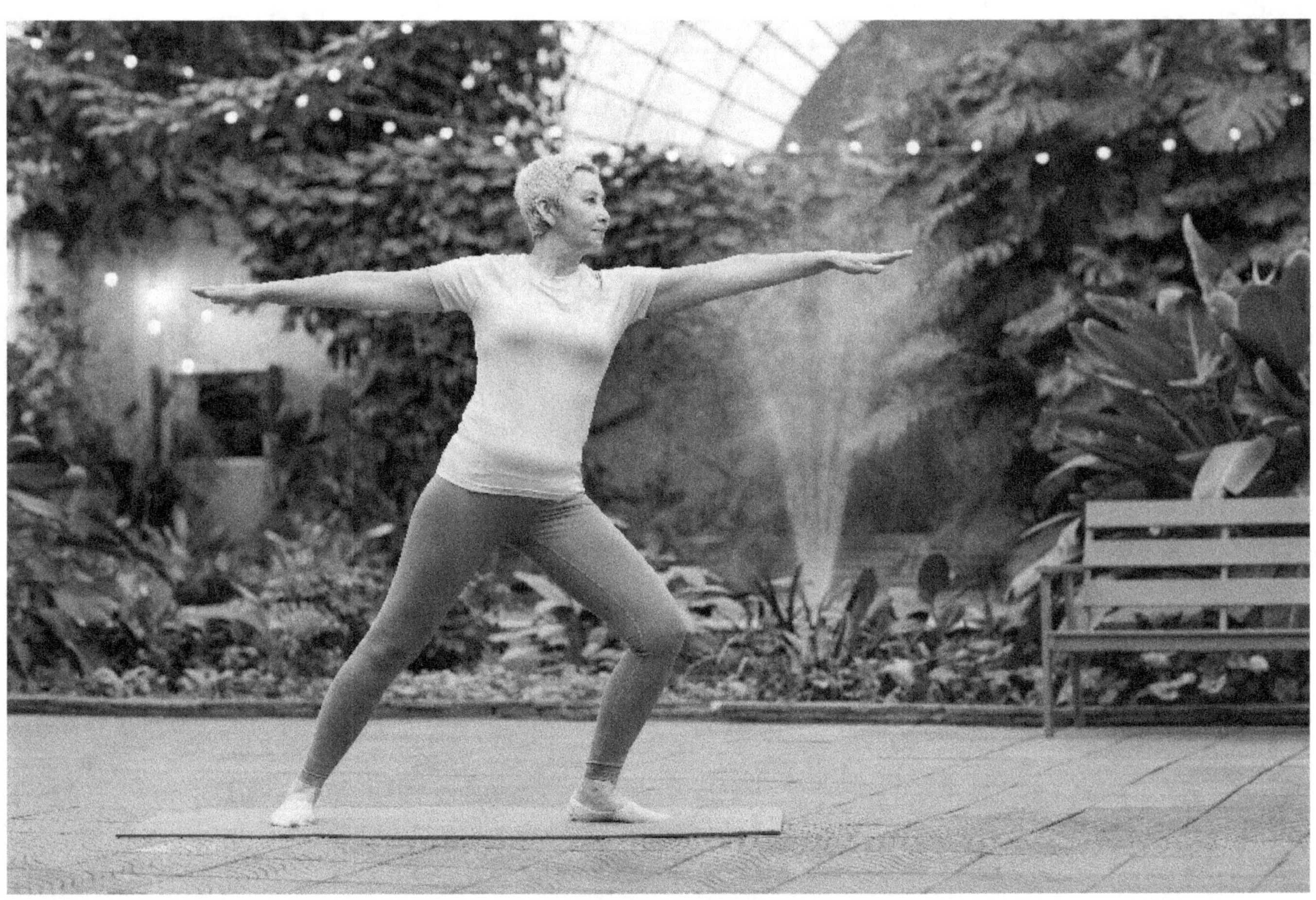

This type of exercise helps build muscle and strength. Examples of strength-training activities include lifting weights, using resistance bands, and doing bodyweight exercises.

Flexibility exercises

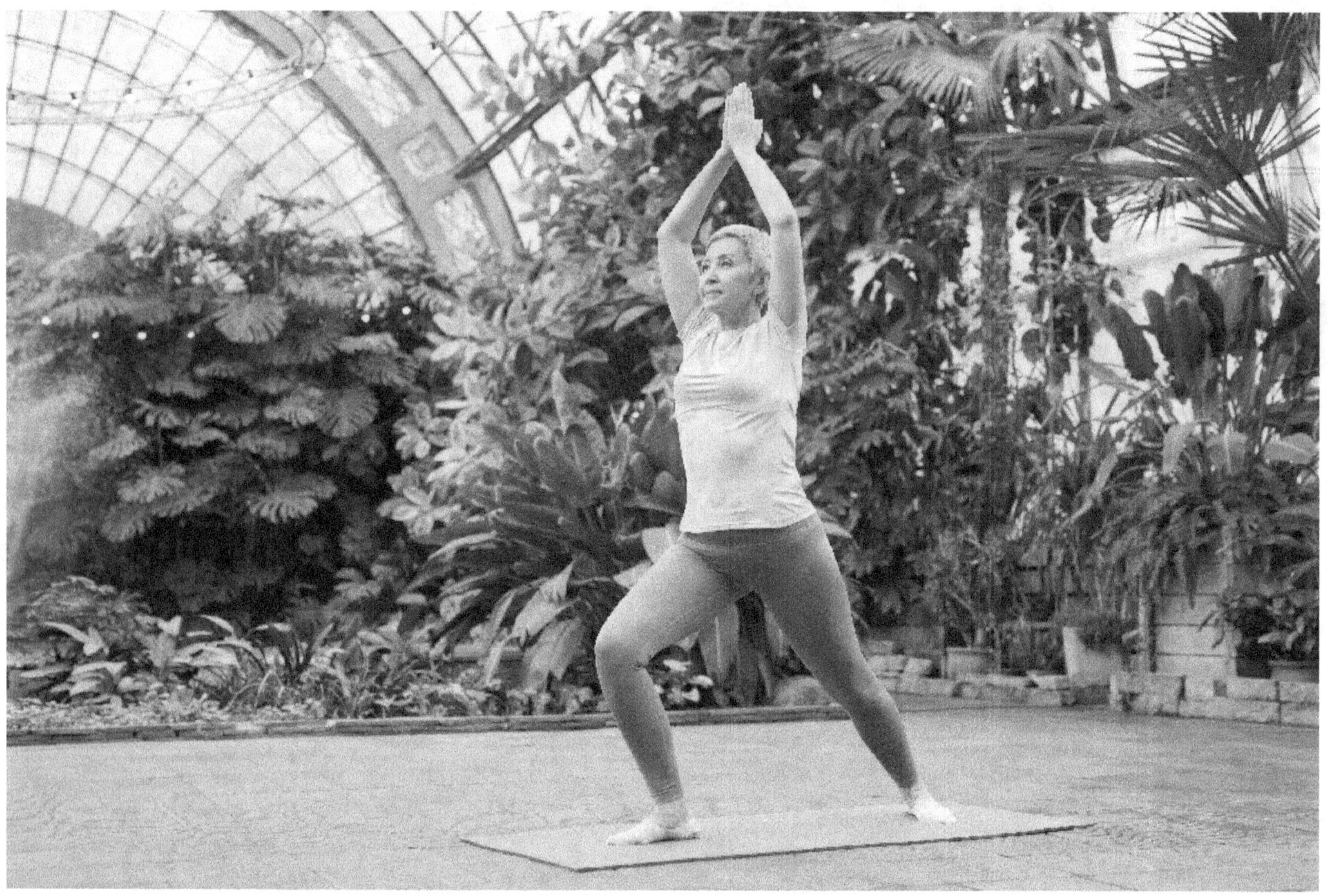

This type of exercise helps improve your range of motion. Examples of flexibility exercises include yoga, Pilates, and tai chi.

Conclusion

Exercise is an essential part of a healthy lifestyle. Following the tips in this chapter, you can find an exercise routine that works for you and improves your overall health.

CHAPTER 3: STRESS MANAGEMENT

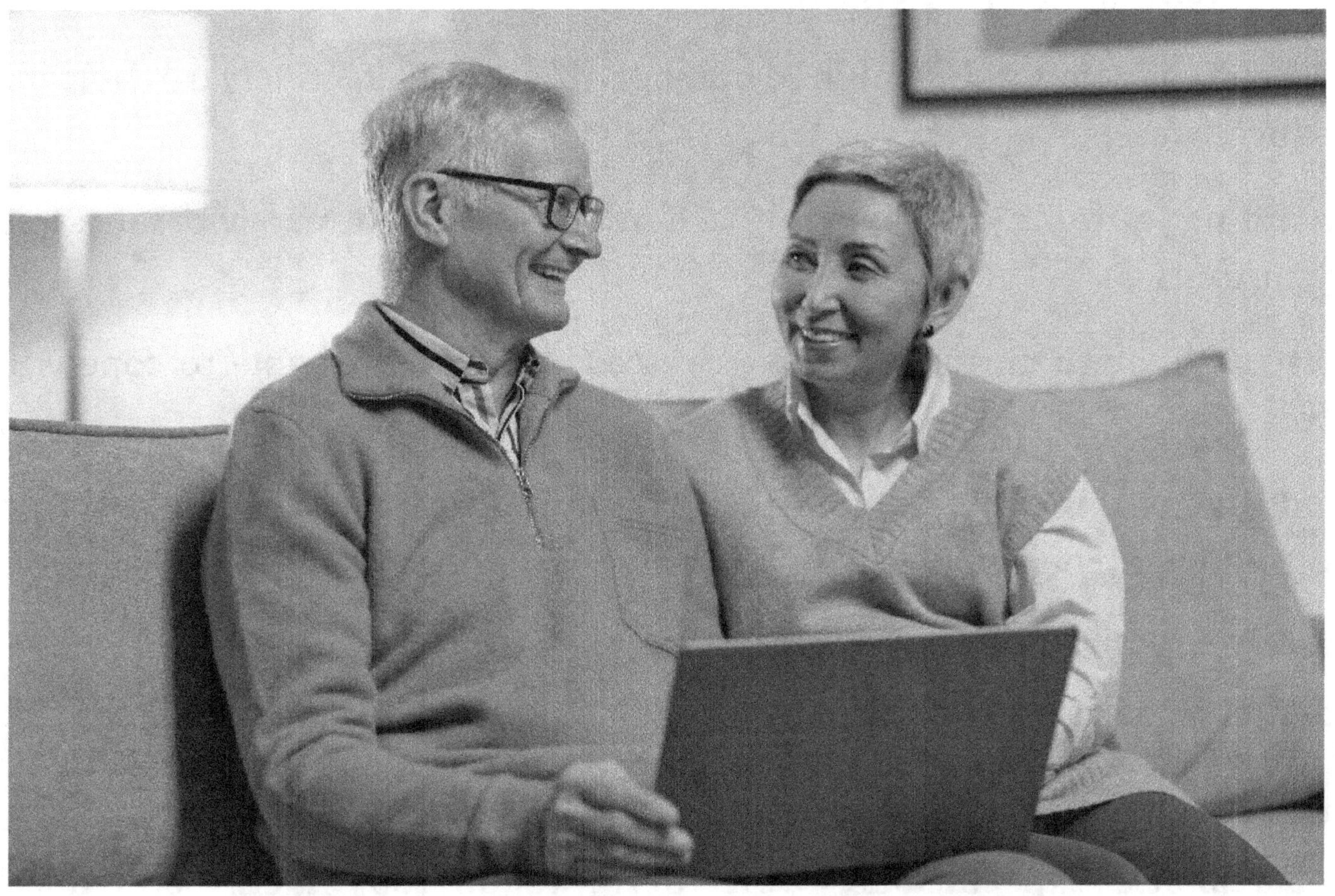

THE IMPORTANCE OF STRESS MANAGEMENT

Stress is a normal part of life, but too much stress can negatively affect your health. Stress can lead to headaches, stomach problems, sleep problems, and even heart disease. It can also make it difficult to concentrate and make decisions.

HOW TO MANAGE STRESS

There are many different ways to manage stress. Some effective techniques include:

Exercise: Exercise is a great way to relieve stress. It releases endorphins, which have mood-boosting effects.

Relaxation techniques: Relaxation techniques, such as deep breathing and meditation, can help you relax.

Time management: Learning to manage your time effectively can help you reduce stress.

Avoiding caffeine and alcohol: Caffeine and alcohol can worsen stress symptoms.

Getting enough sleep: When well-rested, you're better able to cope with stress.

Talking to someone: Talking to a friend, family member, therapist, or counselor can help you deal with stress.

Here are some additional tips for managing stress:

Identify your stressors: The first step to managing stress is to identify the things that are causing you stress. Once you know your stressors, you can start developing coping strategies.

Set realistic expectations: Wait to try to do too much. Set realistic expectations for yourself, and don't hesitate to ask for help when needed.

Take breaks: When you're feeling stressed, take a break from whatever you're doing and do something you enjoy, such as reading, walking, or listening to music.

Reward yourself: When you've successfully managed stress, reward yourself with something you enjoy; this will help you stay motivated and on track.

Conclusion

Remember, stress is a normal part of life, but it doesn't have to control you. Following the tips in this chapter, you can learn how to manage stress and improve your overall health.

CHAPTER 4: SLEEP

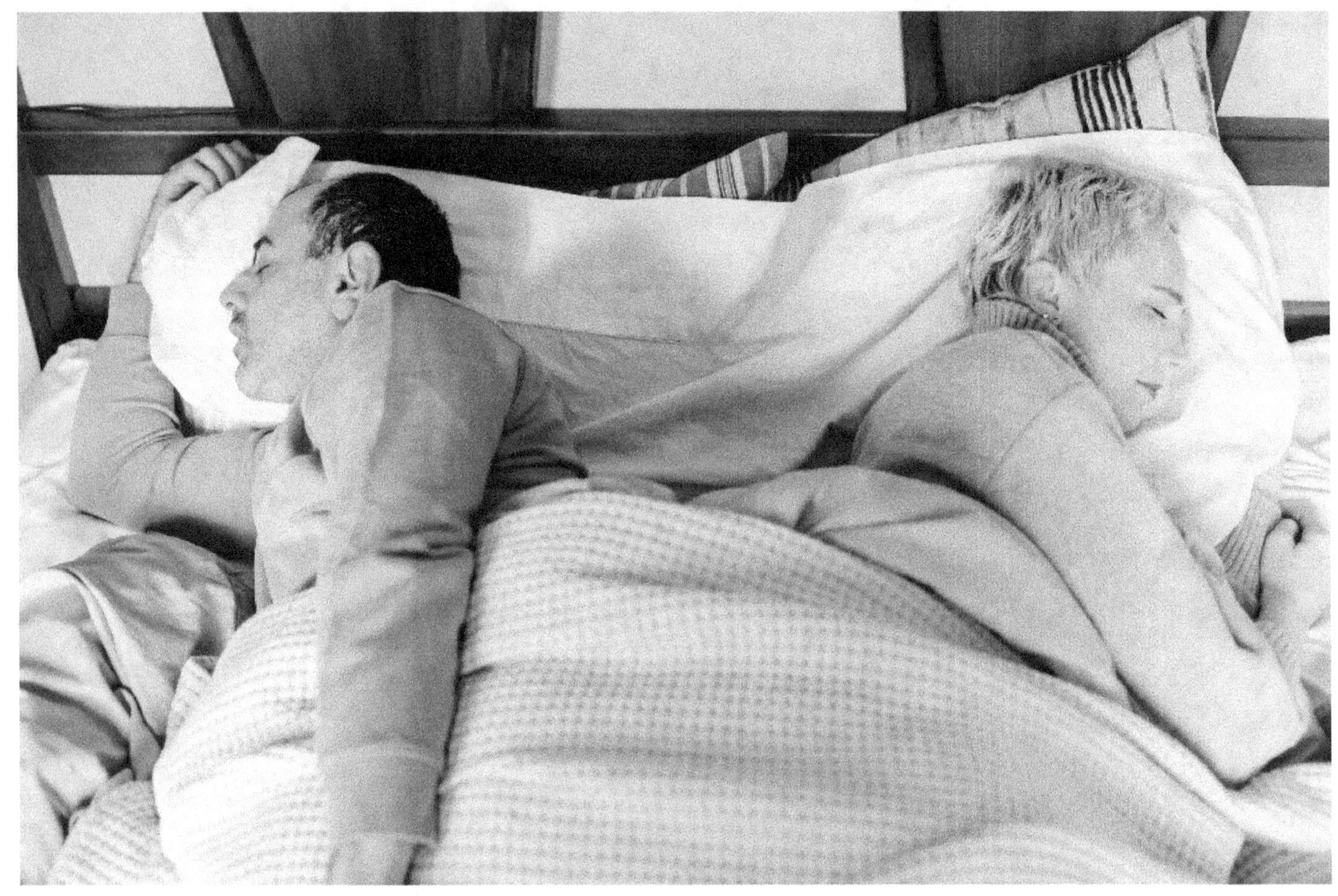

THE IMPORTANCE OF SLEEP

Sleep is essential for good health. It allows your body to rest and repair itself, and it helps you function at your best, both physically and mentally.

How Much Sleep Do You Need?

The amount of sleep you need varies depending on your age. Adults typically require 7-8 hours of sleep per night. However, some people may need more or less sleep.

THE EFFECTS OF SLEEP DEPRIVATION

Sleep deprivation can have several negative consequences for your health, including:

Increased risk of accidents: Sleep-deprived people are more likely to have accidents at work and in everyday life.

Increased risk of chronic diseases: Sleep deprivation can increase your risk of developing chronic diseases such as heart disease, stroke, type 2 diabetes, and obesity.

Decreased cognitive function: Sleep deprivation can impair cognitive function, making it difficult to concentrate, make decisions, and learn new things.

Increased risk of depression: Sleep deprivation can increase your risk of developing depression.

TIPS TO GET A GOOD NIGHT'S SLEEP

Establish a regular sleep schedule: Go to bed and wake up simultaneously each day, even on weekends.

Create a relaxing bedtime routine: Take a warm bath, read a book, or listen to calming music.

Ensure your bedroom is dark, quiet, and calm: These conditions are ideal for sleep.

Avoid caffeine and alcohol before bed: These substances can interfere with sleep.

Get regular exercise: Exercise can help you sleep better at night.

See a doctor if you have trouble sleeping: If you've tried the tips above and you're still having trouble sleeping, talk to your doctor. There may be an underlying medical condition that's interfering with your sleep.

Conclusion

Sleep is essential for good health. Following the tips in this chapter, you can improve your sleep habits and get the rest you need to feel your best.

CHAPTER 5: DRINK WATER

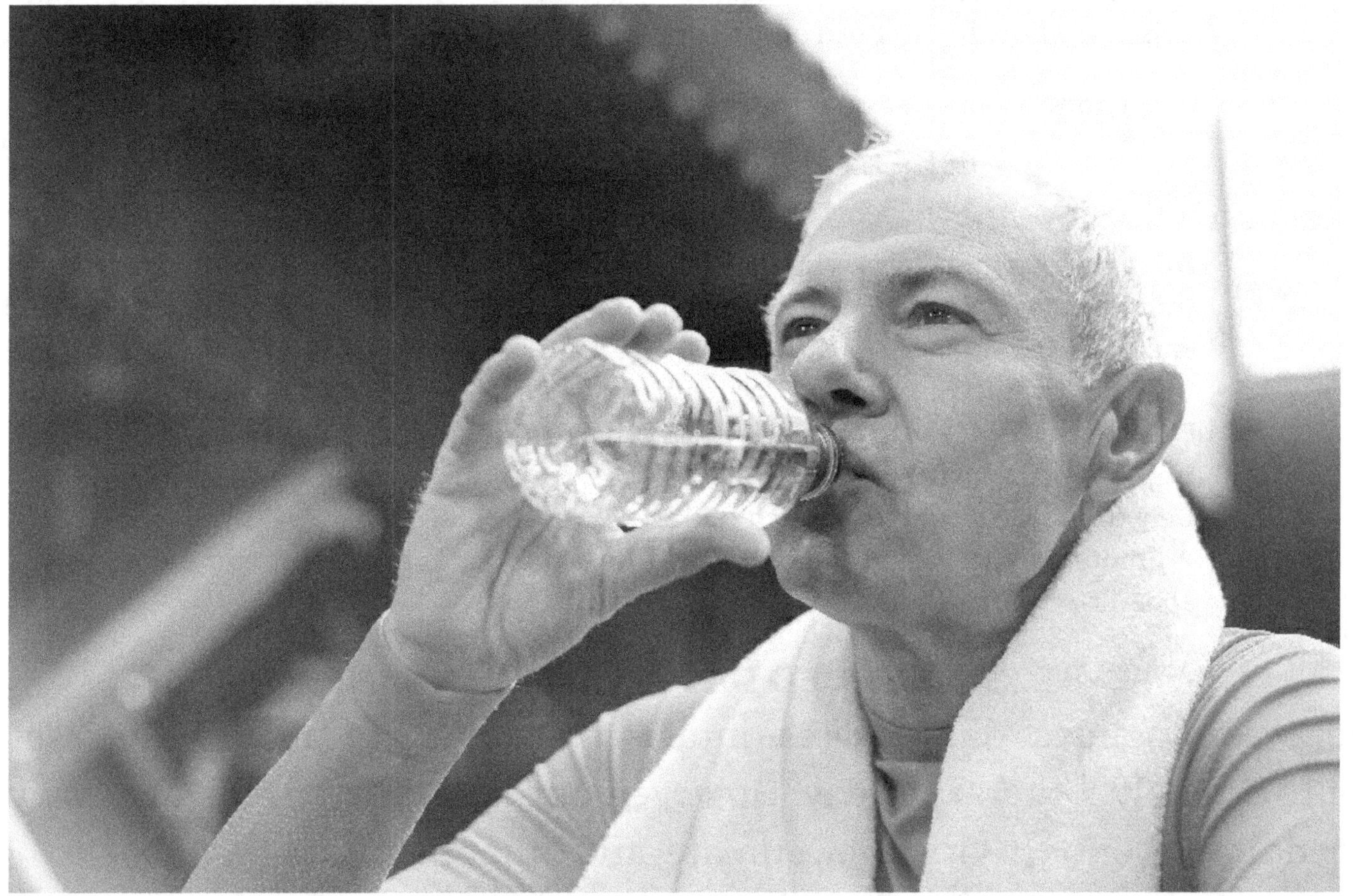

Water is a crucial element for survival. Our body weight consists of 60% water, which plays an important role in many bodily functions. It helps regulate body temperature, deliver nutrients and oxygen to cells, and remove waste materials.

Drinking enough water is important for our overall health and well-being.

WATER CAN HELP TO PREVENT HEALTH PROBLEMS

- **Dehydration:** When we don't drink enough water, our bodies become dehydrated. Experiencing fatigue, headache, dizziness, and constipation are common symptoms that may occur as a result of this condition.
- **Constipation:** Water helps to keep our digestive system running smoothly. If we don't drink enough water, our stools can become hard and difficult to pass.

- **Urinary tract infections (UTIs):** Urinary tract infections (UTIs) are a frequently occurring infection that can impact the bladder, urethra, or kidneys. Drinking water aids in removing bacteria from the urinary tract, thereby reducing the risk of developing UTIs.
- **Kidney stones:** Kidney stones are hard deposits that can form in the kidneys. Water helps to keep the urine dilute, which can help to prevent kidney stones.
- **Headaches:** Headaches can be caused by a number of factors, including dehydration. Drinking enough water can help to prevent headaches or reduce their severity.

WATER CAN HELP TO IMPROVE OUR OVERALL HEALTH AND WELL-BEING

Water can help to:

- **Increase energy levels:** When we're dehydrated, our bodies have to work harder to function, which can lead to fatigue. Drinking enough water can help to boost our energy levels.
- **Improve cognitive function:** Water helps to keep our brains functioning properly. Dehydration can lead to problems with concentration, memory, and decision-making.
- **Improve skin health:** Water helps to keep our skin hydrated and looking its best. Dehydration can lead to dry, itchy skin.
- **Promote weight loss:** Water can help to boost our metabolism and suppress our appetite.

RECOMMENDED DAILY WATER INTAKE

The recommended daily water intake for adults is about 8 glasses (approximately 2 liters) per day. However, our individual needs may vary depending on our activity level, climate, and other factors.

The best way to know if you're drinking enough water is to pay attention to your thirst. If you're feeling thirsty, you're already dehydrated. Aim to drink water before you feel thirsty.

There are a number of ways to make drinking water more enjoyable. You can add flavor to your water with slices of fruit, herbs, or spices. You can also try sparkling water or flavored water.

Drinking enough water is an important part of a healthy lifestyle. By making an effort to drink water throughout the day, you can help to prevent a variety of health problems and improve your overall health and well-being.

WATER DRINKING TIPS

Here are some tips for drinking more water:

- Keep a water bottle with you at all times.
- Set a reminder on your phone to drink water throughout the day.
- Drink water with your meals and snacks.
- Make water your go-to drink when you're thirsty.
- Add flavor to your water with fruit, herbs, or spices.
- Try sparkling water or flavored water.

Remember, water is essential for life. So drink up!

CHAPTER 6: OTHER LIFESTYLE FACTORS

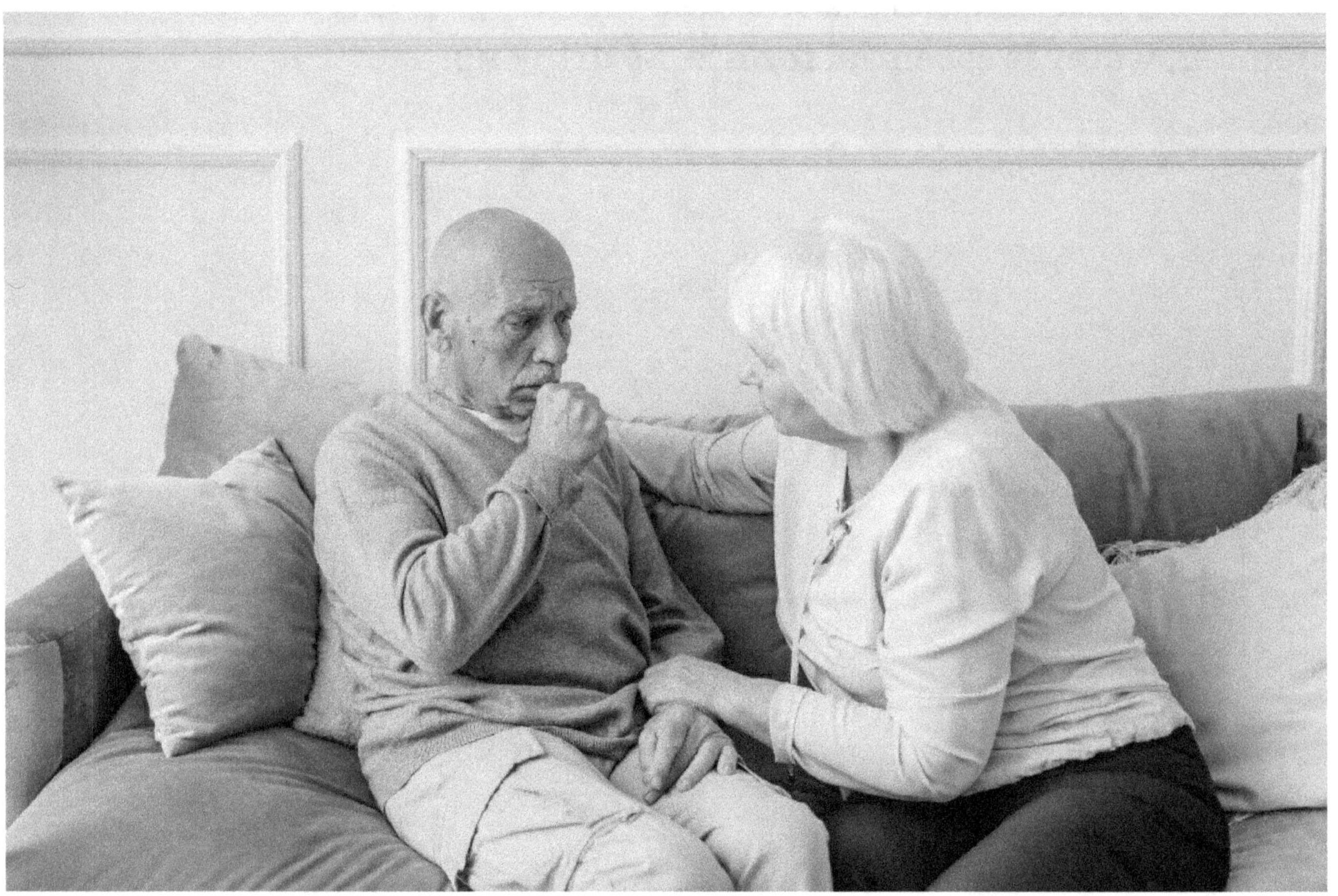

In addition to diet, exercise, stress management, and sleep deprivation, several other lifestyle and environmental factors can affect your health. These include:

Smoking

Smoking is the leading cause of preventable death in the United States. It can increase your risk of developing heart disease, stroke, cancer, and other chronic diseases.

Alcohol use

Excessive alcohol use can damage your liver, heart, and other organs. It can also increase your risk of developing cancer and other health problems.

Sun exposure

Too much sun exposure can increase your risk of developing skin cancer. Wearing sunscreen, sunglasses, and a hat is essential to protect your skin from the sun.

Weight management

Being overweight or obese is a significant risk factor for many chronic diseases, including heart disease, stroke, type 2 diabetes, and some types of cancer.

TIPS FOR MANAGING LIFESTYLE FACTORS THAT AFFECT YOUR HEALTH

Quit smoking:

If you smoke, quitting is the best thing you can do for your health. Many resources are available to help you stop, such as the National Cancer Institute's Smokefree.gov website.

Drink alcohol in moderation:

If you drink alcohol, do so in moderation. The Centers for Disease Control and Prevention (CDC) recommends that women have no more than one drink per day and men have no more than two drinks per day.

Protect your skin from the sun:

Wear sunscreen with an SPF of 30 or higher daily, even on cloudy days. You should also wear sunglasses and a hat to protect your face and neck from the sun.

Maintain a healthy weight:

If you're overweight or obese, talk to your doctor about how to lose weight safely. There are many ways to lose weight, such as diet, exercise, and behavior modification.

Get regular screening tests:

Talk to your doctor about which screening tests are proper for you. These tests can help detect diseases early when they're most treatable.

Conclusion

Many lifestyle and environmental factors can affect your health. By making healthy choices in these areas, following the tips in this chapter can improve your health and reduce your risk of developing chronic diseases.

CHAPTER 7: SCREENING TESTS

Screening tests are used to detect diseases early when they're most treatable. Many screening tests, such as mammograms, colonoscopies, and blood pressure checks, are recommended for adults.

BENEFITS OF SCREENING TESTS

Early detection: Screening tests can help detect diseases when they're most treatable. This can lead to better outcomes and longer life.

Prevention: In some cases, screening tests can help prevent diseases from developing. For example, if you have high blood pressure, you can take steps to lower it and reduce your risk of developing heart disease or stroke.

Peace of mind: Screening tests can give you peace of mind knowing that you're doing everything possible to stay healthy.

THE RISKS OF SCREENING TESTS

False positives: A false positive is when a screening test shows that you have a disease but don't. This can lead to unnecessary anxiety and further testing.

False negatives: A false negative is when a screening test shows that you don't have a disease but actually do. This can lead to delays in diagnosis and treatment.

The decision of whether or not to have a screening test is a personal one. You should talk to your doctor about the benefits and risks of each test and decide what's right for you.

COMMON SCREENING TESTS RECOMMENDED FOR ADULTS

Mammogram: A mammogram is a low-dose X-ray of the breasts that can help detect breast cancer early.

Colonoscopy: A colonoscopy is a procedure that uses a long, thin tube with a camera to examine the inside of the colon and rectum. This test can help detect colon cancer and polyps, which can develop into cancer.

Blood pressure check: A blood pressure check is a simple test that can help detect high blood pressure, a major risk factor for heart disease and stroke.

Cholesterol screening: A cholesterol screening is a test that measures the levels of cholesterol in your blood. High cholesterol is a major risk factor for heart disease and stroke.

Pap smear: A Pap smear is a test that can help detect cervical cancer.

Flu shot: The flu shot is a vaccine that can help protect you from the flu.

Conclusion
These are just a few of the many available screening tests. Talk to your doctor about which tests are right for you.

CHAPTER 8: PYRAMID ENERGY MAT

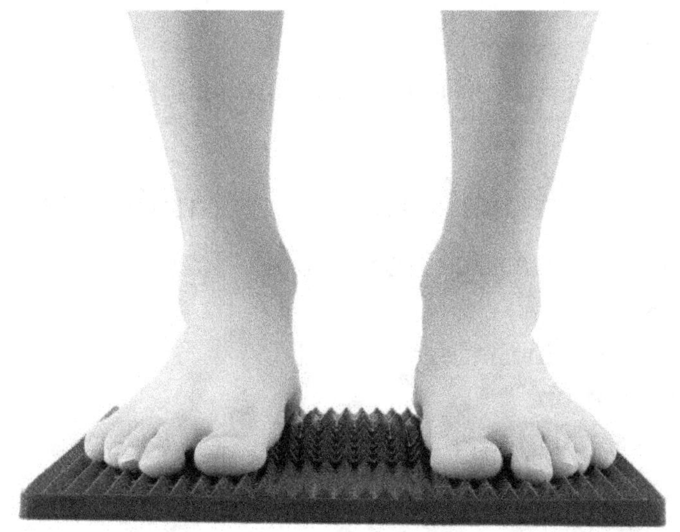

WHAT IS PYRAMID ENERGY MAT?

The pyramid energy mat uses acupressure and magnetic therapy to promote health and well-being. Acupressure is an ancient Chinese healing technique that involves applying pressure to specific points on the body. Magnetic therapy is the use of magnets to promote healing.

HOW DOES IT WORK?

When you step on a pyramid energy mat, the acupressure points on the soles of your feet are stimulated. These benefits are improving blood circulation, reducing stress, and relieving pain. The magnets in the mat also help to improve circulation and promote healing.

EFFECTS OF USING PYRAMID ENERGY MAT

Regular use of a pyramid energy mat can help prevent various health problems. For example, it can help to:

- Reduce stress and anxiety
- Improve sleep quality
- Relieve pain from headaches, muscle aches, and arthritis
- Improve digestion
- Boost the immune system
- Reduce the risk of heart disease, stroke, and diabetes

In addition to its preventive benefits, the pyramid energy mat can also care for various existing health conditions. For example, it can be used to:

- Relieve back pain
- Improve circulation in the legs
- Reduce inflammation
- Treat headaches and migraines
- Improve mood
- Boost energy levels

The pyramid energy mat may be a good option if you are looking for a natural way to improve your health and well-being. *However, it is important to note that the pyramid energy mat is not a cure-all. It is important to consult with a doctor if you have any serious health conditions.*

TIPS FOR USING A PYRAMID ENERGY MAT FOR PREVENTION

- Start with short sessions and gradually increase the amount of time you spend on the mat each day.
- If you have any pain, stop using the mat immediately.
- If you are pregnant, consult with your doctor before using the mat.
- Keep the mat clean and dry.

CHAPTER 9: ALKALINE IN THE BODY

The human body is naturally slightly alkaline, with a blood pH of around 7.4. This means the body's fluids are slightly basic, unlike acidic. Alkaline fluids are important for maintaining a healthy immune system, preventing disease, and promoting overall well-being.

SUPPLEMENTS AND LIFESTYLE CHANGES TO KEEP THE BODY ALKALINE

- **Eating an alkaline diet:** This means eating plenty of fruits, vegetables, and whole grains and avoiding processed foods, sugary drinks, and red meat.

- **Drinking alkaline water:** Alkaline water is water that has been infused with minerals, such as calcium, magnesium, and potassium. These minerals help to alkalize the body's fluids.

- **Taking alkaline supplements:** There are a number of alkaline supplements available, such as baking soda, potassium bicarbonate, and magnesium oxide. These supplements can help to alkalize the body's fluids and promote overall health.

In addition to these dietary and supplement changes, there are a number of other lifestyle habits that can help to keep the body alkaline, such as:

- **Getting regular exercise:** Exercise helps to remove toxins from the body and promote circulation.

- **Getting enough sleep:** Sleep is essential for the body's natural detoxification processes.

- **Managing stress:** Stress can lead to an acidic pH in the body. Managing stress through relaxation techniques, such as yoga or meditation, can help to keep the body alkaline.

By following these tips, you can help to keep your body alkaline and prevent common health problems.

BENEFITS OF KEEPING THE BODY ALKALINE

- **Improved digestion:** Alkaline fluids help to break down food and absorb nutrients.

- **Reduced inflammation:** Inflammation is a major factor in many chronic diseases. Alkaline fluids help to reduce inflammation and promote healing.

- **Enhanced energy levels:** Alkaline fluids help to provide the body with energy.

- **Improved skin health:** Alkaline fluids help to keep the skin looking healthy and radiant.

CHAPTER 10: HEALTHY MID-AGE FOODS BY CONTINENT

These are just a few examples of food that is recommended for mid-age people in each continent, the recommendation is based on available foods and fruits common in each location at large. It is important to choose a variety of foods from all food groups to ensure that you are getting all the nutrients you need.

Please note that the availability of food in each continent can vary depending on the time of year and the location, It is important to note that some traditional foods can be high in calories and fat. so be mindful of portion sizes and to choose healthier cooking methods, such as grilling, baking, or steaming. It is also important to consult with a doctor or registered dietitian to create a personalized meal plan that meets your individual needs.

TIPS FOR EATING A HEALTHY DIET IN MID-AGE AND ABOVE

- **Eat plenty of fruits and vegetables.** Fruits and vegetables are low in calories and fat and high in vitamins, minerals, and fiber. They can help you feel full and satisfied, which can help you maintain a healthy weight.
- **Choose lean protein sources.** Lean protein sources include fish, chicken, beans, and tofu. They are low in saturated fat and calories and high in protein.
- **Limit unhealthy fats.** Unhealthy fats, such as saturated and trans fats, can raise your cholesterol levels and increase your risk of heart disease. Limit your intake

of unhealthy fats by choosing lean protein sources, cooking with healthy oils, and avoiding processed foods.

- **Eat whole grains.** Whole grains are a good source of fiber, vitamins, and minerals. They can help you feel full and satisfied, which can help you maintain a healthy weight.
- **Stay hydrated.** Drinking plenty of water is important for overall health. It can help you feel full and satisfied, and it can also help your body function properly.

Following these tips can help you eat a healthy diet in mid-age and support your overall health and well-being.

RECOMMENDED MID-AGE FOOD BY CONTINENT

AFRICA

- **Beans:** Beans are an excellent source of protein, fiber, and iron. They also contain complex carbohydrates that can help you feel full and satisfied.
- **Fish:** Fish is a good source of protein, omega-3 fatty acids, and vitamin D. Omega-3 fatty acids are important for heart health and cognitive function.
- **Nuts and seeds:** Nuts and seeds are a good source of protein, fiber, and healthy fats. Foods like these provide essential nutrients like magnesium, phosphorus, and zinc, which are important for maintaining a healthy body.
- **Vegetables:** Vegetables are a good source of vitamins, minerals, and fiber. They are also low in calories and fat.
- **Fruits:** Fruits provide essential vitamins, minerals, and fiber while having low calorie and fat content.

Traditional dishes: There are a few traditional dishes in Africa that are good for mid-age people and above. Some examples include:

- **Egusi soup:** A Nigerian soup made with ground melon seeds, spinach, and meat. It is a good source of protein, fiber, and vitamins A and C.
- **Fufu:** A West African dish made with pounded cassava or plantain. It is often served with soups or stews. It is a good source of complex carbohydrates and fiber.
- **Suya:** A skewered meat that is grilled or roasted. It is often seasoned with chili peppers and spices. It is a good source of protein and iron.
- **Tindouf couscous:** A couscous dish from Algeria that is made with semolina, vegetables, and lamb or beef. It is a good source of complex carbohydrates, fiber, and protein.

- **Lentil soup:** A soup made with lentils, tomatoes, and spices. It is a good source of protein, fiber, and iron.
- **Mashed sweet potatoes:** Mashed sweet potatoes are a good source of beta-carotene, vitamin C, and fiber.
- **African eggplant stew:** A stew made with eggplant, tomatoes, and spices. It is a good source of fiber, potassium, and vitamin C.
- **Jollof rice:** A rice dish that is popular in West Africa. It is made with rice, tomatoes, onions, and spices. It is a good source of complex carbohydrates, fiber, and vitamin C.

ANTARCTICA

- **Fresh seafood:** Fresh seafood is a good source of protein, omega-3 fatty acids, and vitamin D. Omega-3 fatty acids are important for heart health and cognitive function. Some popular fresh seafood in Antarctica include fish, squid, and krill.
- **MRE:** Meals Ready to Eat (MREs) are a good source of nutrients and calories. They are also a good option for people who are on the go or who do not have access to fresh food.
- **Dried fruits and vegetables:** Dried fruits and vegetables are a good source of vitamins, minerals, and fiber. They are also a good option for people who are on the go or who do not have access to fresh food.
- **Nuts and seeds:** Nuts and seeds are a good source of protein, fiber, and healthy fats. They are also a good source of vitamins and minerals, such as magnesium, phosphorus, and zinc.

Traditional dishes: There are a few traditional dishes in Antarctica that are good for mid-age people and above. Some examples include:

- **Hoosh:** A stew made with meat, vegetables, and grains.
- **Pemmican:** A mixture of dried meat, fat, and berries.
- **Sledging biscuits:** Hard biscuits that are high in calories and nutrients.

ASIA

- **Tofu:** Tofu is a good source of protein, calcium, and iron. It is also a good source of isoflavones, which have been shown to have health benefits, such as reducing the risk of heart disease and cancer.
- **Edamame:** Edamame is soybeans that are steamed or boiled. They are a good source of protein, fiber, and is of lavones.
- **Tempeh:** Tempeh is a fermented soybean product. It is a good source of protein, fiber, and iron. It is also a good source of probiotics, which are beneficial bacteria for the gut.
- **Brown rice:** Brown rice is a whole grain that is a good source of fiber, vitamins, and minerals. It is also a good source of antioxidants.
- **Vegetables:** Vegetables are a good source of vitamins, minerals, and fiber. They are also low in calories and fat.

Traditional dishes: There are a few traditional dishes in Asia that are good for mid-age people and above. Some examples include:

Fruits: Fruits are a good source of vitamins, minerals, and fiber. They are also low in calories and fat.

- **Soup:** Soup is a good way to get your daily dose of vegetables and protein. It is also a filling meal that can help you feel full.
- **Noodles:** Noodles are a good source of carbohydrates, which can give you energy. *They can also be a good source of protein and fiber, depending on the type of noodles you choose.*

EUROPE

- **Olive oil:** Olive oil is a good source of healthy fats, such as monounsaturated fats. Monounsaturated fats are important for heart health.
- **Salmon:** Salmon is a good source of protein, omega-3 fatty acids, and vitamin D.

Omega-3 fatty acids are important for heart health and cognitive function.
- **Yogurt:** Yogurt is a good source of protein, calcium, and probiotics. Probiotics are beneficial bacteria for the gut.
- **Green leafy vegetables:** Green leafy vegetables are a good source of vitamins, minerals, and fiber. They are also low in calories and fat.
- **Fruits:** Fruits are a good source of vitamins, minerals, and fiber. They are also low in calories and fat.

Traditional dishes: There are a few traditional dishes in Europe that are good for mid-age people and above. Some examples include:

- **Gazpacho:** A cold soup made from tomatoes, cucumbers, onions, and garlic. It is a good source of vitamins C and K, as well as lycopene.
- **Hummus:** A dip or spread made from mashed chickpeas, tahini, lemon juice, and garlic. It is a good source of protein, fiber, and healthy fats.
- **Lentil soup:** Lentil soup is a good source of protein, fiber, and iron. It is also a good source of vitamins A and C.
- **Roasted vegetables:** Roasted vegetables are a good source of vitamins, minerals, and fiber. They are also a good source of antioxidants.
- **Whole-wheat pasta:** Whole-wheat pasta is a good source of complex carbohydrates, fiber, and protein. It is also a good source of iron.

NORTH AMERICA

- **Black Beans:** Beans are a good source of protein, fiber, and iron. They are also a good source of complex carbohydrates, which can help you feel full and satisfied.
- **Salmon:** Salmon is a good source of protein, omega-3 fatty acids, and vitamin D. Omega-3 fatty acids are important for heart health and cognitive function.
- **Olive oil:** Olive oil is a good source of healthy fats, such as monounsaturated fats. Monounsaturated fats are important for heart health.
- **Vegetables:** Vegetables are a good source of vitamins, minerals, and fiber. They are also low in calories and fat.
- **Fruits:** Fruits are a good source of vitamins, minerals, and fiber. They are also low in calories and fat.

Traditional dishes: There are a few traditional dishes in North America that are good for mid-age people and above. Some examples include:

- **Quinoa:** A whole grain that is a good source of protein, fiber, and iron. It is also a good source of antioxidants.

- **Oatmeal:** A whole grain that is a good source of fiber, vitamins, and minerals. It is also a good source of complex carbohydrates, which can help you feel full and satisfied.
- **Lentil soup:** A soup made with lentils, tomatoes, and spices. It is a good source of protein, fiber, and iron.
- **Roasted vegetables:** Roasted vegetables are a good source of vitamins, minerals, and fiber. They are also low in calories and fat.
- **Fruit salad:** A fruit salad is a good source of vitamins, minerals, and fiber. It is also a low-calorie snack or dessert option.
- **Hummus:** A dip made from chickpeas, tahini, lemon juice, and garlic. It is a good source of protein, fiber, and healthy fats.

OCEANIA

- **Fish:** Fish is a good source of protein, omega-3 fatty acids, and vitamin D. Omega-3 fatty acids are important for heart health and cognitive function. Some popular fish in Oceania include salmon, tuna, mackerel, and sardines.
- **Fruits and vegetables:** Fruits and vegetables are a good source of vitamins, minerals, and fiber. They are also low in calories and fat. Some popular fruits and vegetables in Oceania include bananas, papayas, mangoes, sweet potatoes, and leafy greens.
- **Whole grains:** Whole grains are a good source of fiber, vitamins, and minerals. They are also a good source of complex carbohydrates, which can help you feel full and satisfied. Some popular whole grains in Oceania include taro, yams, quinoa, and brown rice.
- **Legumes:** Legumes are a good source of protein, fiber, and iron. They are also a good source of complex carbohydrates, which can help you feel full and satisfied. Some popular legumes in Oceania include lentils, beans, and chickpeas.
- **Nuts and seeds:** Nuts and seeds are a good source of protein, fiber, and healthy fats. They are also a good source of vitamins and minerals, such as magnesium, phosphorus, and zinc. Some popular nuts and seeds in Oceania include almonds, walnuts, and sunflower seeds.

Traditional dishes: There are many traditional dishes in Oceania that are good for mid-age people and above. Some examples include:

- **Lakatan:** A Filipino dish made with coconut milk, young coconut meat, and tapioca pearls.
- **Puka puka:** A Samoan dish made with taro leaves, coconut milk, and fish.
- **Kalua pork:** A Hawaiian dish made with pork shoulder that is slow-cooked in an underground oven.
- **Miso soup:** A Japanese dish made with miso paste, dashi broth, and various toppings.

SOUTH AMERICA

- **Quinoa:** Quinoa is a whole grain that is a good source of protein, magnesium, fiber, and iron. It can be eaten as a side dish, in salads, or used to make veggie burgers, It is also a good source of antioxidants.
- **Lentils:** Lentils are a good source of protein, fiber, and iron. They can be cooked in a variety of ways, such as in soups, stews, or salads. They are also a good source of complex carbohydrates, which can help you feel full and satisfied.
- **Brazil nuts:** Brazil nuts are a good source of selenium, which is an important mineral for the body.
- **Acai berries:** Acai berries are high in antioxidants and fiber. It can be eaten fresh, frozen, or as a juice, it can help protect the body from damage.

Traditional dishes: There are many traditional dishes in South America that are good for mid-age people and above. Some examples include:

- **Hummus:** A dip made from chickpeas, tahini, lemon juice, and garlic. It is a good source of protein and fiber.
- **Guacamole:** A dip made from avocados, tomatoes, onions, and cilantro. It is a good source of healthy fats, fiber, and potassium.
- **Ceviche:** A dish of raw fish that is cured in citrus juice. It is a good source of protein and omega-3 fatty acids.
- **Empanadas:** A pastry filled with meat, cheese, or vegetables. They are a good source of carbohydrates, protein, and fiber.
- **Yuca:** A root vegetable that is high in carbohydrates and fiber. It can be boiled, mashed,

or fried.

CHAPTER 11: OVERALL WELLNESS

There are many different types of wellness, but some of the most common include:

Physical wellness: This refers to your overall physical health, including your fitness level, nutrition, and sleep habits.

Emotional wellness: This refers to your mental health and emotional well-being. It includes managing stress, coping with difficult emotions, and maintaining a positive outlook.

Social wellness: This refers to your relationships with others. It includes your ability to connect with others, build strong relationships, and feel supported by your community.

Intellectual wellness refers to your cognitive health and ability to learn and grow. It includes your curiosity, creativity, and ability to solve problems.

Spiritual wellness refers to your sense of purpose and meaning in life. It includes your connection to a greater being than yourself and your ability to find peace and happiness.

These are just a few of the many different types of wellness. It is important to find a balance between all of these areas to achieve overall wellness.

IMPROVING YOUR WELLNESS

- **Physical wellness:** Eat a healthy diet, exercise regularly, and get enough sleep.
- **Emotional wellness:** Find healthy stress management methods, such as exercise, yoga, or meditation. Spend time with loved ones, do things you enjoy, and practice self-care.
- **Social wellness:** Connect with others, build strong relationships, and get involved in your community.
- **Intellectual wellness:** Challenge yourself, learn new things, and stay curious.
- **Spiritual wellness:** Find something that gives your life meaning and purpose. Spend

time in nature, connect with your religious community, or meditate and reflect on your life.

CHAPTER 12: CONCLUSION

Prevention is the key to good health.

By making healthy choices in your diet, exercise, stress management, sleep, and other lifestyle factors, you can reduce your risk of developing chronic diseases and improve your overall health.

Screening tests can also help detect diseases early when they are most treatable. Talk to your doctor about which screening tests are right for you. Taking care of your health is an investment in your future. By making healthy choices today, you can enjoy a longer, healthier, and happier life.

Here are some final tips for staying healthy:

Make healthy choices a habit: The more you make healthy choices, the easier they will become.

Remember to ask for help: Talk to your doctor or a registered dietitian if you struggle to make healthy changes.

Be patient: It takes time to make lasting changes to your health. Keep going even if you don't see results immediately.

Celebrate your successes: When you make a healthy choice, take a moment to celebrate your success. This will help you stay motivated.

Remember, you're not alone: Millions of people are working to improve their health. By making healthy choices and caring for yourself, you can join them and live a long, healthy, and happy life.

Prevention is the key to good health. Following the tips in this book can reduce your risk of developing chronic diseases and improve your overall health.

ABOUT AUTHOR

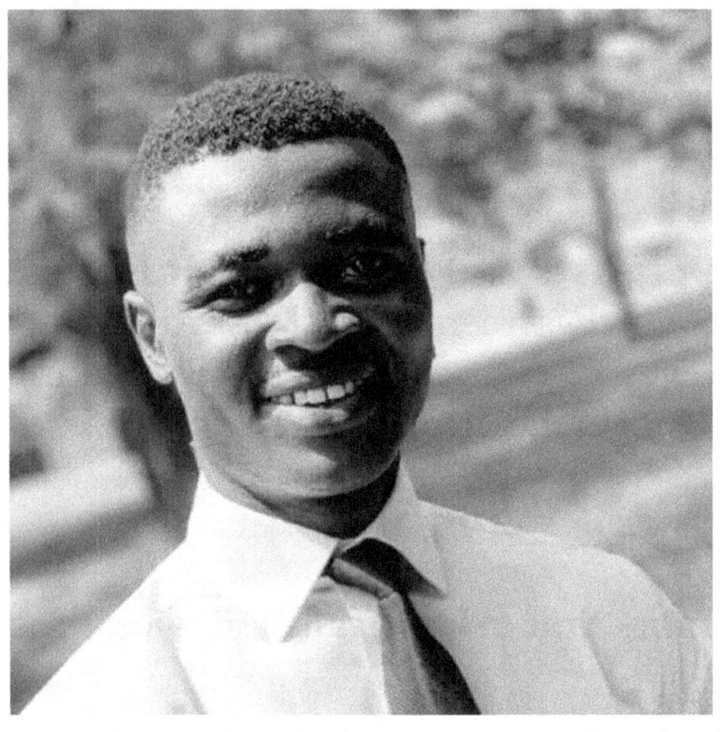

Joseph Rutherford is a Behavioral Change Communicator, a Health and Wellness enthusiast, Digital Marketing Professional, Public Speaker, and Blockchain and Cryptocurrency Enthusiast. He is passionate about helping people live healthier lives and believes prevention is the best medicine.

In this book, "Power of Prevention," Joseph Rutherford shares his knowledge and expertise on protecting yourself and your loved ones from disease while staying healthy and active as you age.

Joseph Rutherford is passionate about helping people live healthier lives. He believes prevention is the best medicine and is committed to providing his audience with the information they need to make healthy choices and behavioral changes.

In addition to his work as an author, Joseph Rutherford is also a frequent public speaker on health and wellness topics. He has helped many people in mid-age and beyond to make informed decisions and lifestyle changes with excellent positive outcomes in their health.

Joseph Rutherford is a strong advocate for preventive care, and he believes that everyone has the right to be healthy. He is committed to helping people make healthy choices and is passionate about empowering people to take control of their health.

"Power of Prevention" covers various topics, including diet and nutrition, exercise, sleep, stress management, and more. Joseph Rutherford also provides practical tips you can implement today.

"Power of Prevention" is a must-read for anyone wanting to live healthier. It's packed with valuable information that can help you reduce your risk of disease and improve the overall health of yourself and your loved ones.

Connect with the Author at:

www.josephrutherford.com

ojosephrutherford@gmail.com

REFERENCES

Harshman, M. (2014, March 17). "You're never too old to get started." Columbian, D.1.

https://universalbloger.com/the-mediterranean-diet-an-amazing-guide-to-a-healthy-lifestyle/

https://issuu.com/rickdelarosa/docs/hmt_dec_2020__2_

https://original.newsbreak.com/@nick-davies-561395/2969683219933-exercise-the-secret-to-a-happy-and-healthy-life

https://www.drshillingford.com/blog/1-reason-you-need-to-strength-train-for-weight-loss-6006.html

www.fitmotherproject.com

www.mondaycampaigns.org

https://www.blubbs.com/the-benefits-of-moderate-alcohol-consumption-how-to-drink-responsibly.html

https://www.jyfs.org/how-many-cardio-minutes-per-week/

https://bludwing.net/the-benefits-of-exercise-for-overall-health/

https://www.srihatech.com/healthy-lifestyle/try-some-easy-and-important-regular-exercise-for-fitness/

www.lybrate.com

https://www.srihatech.com/healthy-lifestyle/try-some-easy-and-important-regular-exercise-for-fitness/

https://blog.smarthealthshop.com/2023/03/24/lose-weight-gain-confidence-transforming-your-body-and-mind/

https://bliev.com/blogs/news/starting-your-fitness-journey-a-beginner-s-guide

https://weightlosstipsforyou.net/health-benefits-of-exercise/

https://www.pwndigital.com/2023/05/Effective-Tips-for-Achieving-Sustainable-Weight-Loss-224.html

https://www.onehealth.sg/2023/04/05/why-regular-exercise-is-vital-for-your-health-and-well-being/

https://alkasharma.co.in/importance-of-exercise-for-kids/

https://www.healthandfitnessplace.com/tips-and-tricks-for-coping-with-stress-in-the-workplace/

https://www.health-livening.com/busting-stress-stress-management-lesson-plans/

https://y2be.net/how-to-manage-stress-when-youre-a-busy-software-engineer/

https://www.schizophrenic.nyc/fear-not-dont-let-trauma-hold-you-back-anymore/

https://gratefulearthcoffee.com/blogs/coffee/10-proven-ways-to-manage-stress

https://mindfulmotherhood.co/mindful-parenting-for-adhd/

https://brainelevate.com/does-adhd-cause-stress/

https://www.greatdiplomas.com/post/stress-management-and-coping-skills-college-major-description-job-guide/

https://fireflies.ai/blog/5-communication-styles
https://theinspire1coach.com/is-21-days-enough-time-to-change-a-habit
www.cdc.gov
http://www.atlantadunia.com/dunia/health/Articledetail.aspx?q=23
https://issuu.com/crossroadsnews/docs/jun1116
https://www.bbntimes.com/science/scientifically-proven-ways-to-overcome-mental-health-troubles
https://habit4success.com/11-small-changes-you-can-make-to-improve-your-lifestyle/
https://www.fitwirr.com/workout/exercises-for-sciatica/
https://project-expat.com/vendors/english-speaking-fitness-studio-frankfurt/
https://aquacarephysicaltherapy.com/service/fit-for-life-weight-management/
https://www.spineo.org/topics/acupressure/
https://smartstartga.org/new-study-again-finds-mediterranean-diet/
https://www.budgetandthebees.com/how-to-heal-after-a-divorce/
https://nanaseasoning.com/faq.html
https://www.themilkcleanse.com/blogs/reference-guide/how-to-treat-menopause-brain-fog
https://www.vigyanveda.com/blogs/english/sinusitis
https://www.wardvilleworkouts.com/post/4-tips-on-how-to-maintain-a-healthy-heart
https://howtofeedyourfamily.com/thrive-diet